Homemade Lip Balm

A Complete Beginner's Guide to Natural DIY Lip Balms You Can Make Today

Jane Aniston

__Introduction__

I want to thank you and congratulate you for choosing to download the book, *"Homemade Lip Balm - A Complete Beginner's Guide to Natural DIY Lip Balms You Can Make Today"*.

This book contains all the information you need to know in order to start making your own natural, chemical-free lip balms at home today. The ingredients used to make these lip balms are cheap and easily available and the process of making them couldn't be simpler!

In this book we'll cover the differences between homemade lip balms and store-bought lip balms and show you why you really should ditch the expensive, toxic, store-bought variety and start making your own natural, healthy, chemical-free alternatives at home.

This book also includes 22 lip balm recipes. Each recipe will list the ingredients required to make the lip balm and then guide you through the process of exactly what you'll need to do, with simple, easy to follow, step by step instructions, meaning you can be making your own lip balms in no time at all!

Once you feel how soothing natural homemade lip balms are, you'll never want to go back to the harmful, store-bought variety, which can be toxic to not only your body but also the environment.

Thank you again for downloading this book. I hope you enjoy it!

Jane Aniston

Table of contents

Conclusion

A message from the author, Jane Aniston

Chapter 1

Why you should stop using store-bought lip balms and start making your own at home!

Our lips are very sensitive as the skin which covers them is very thin in comparison to most other parts of the body. Since the lips are continuously exposed to heat, cold and other elements, they dry and crack easily. This drying and cracking tends to happen more frequently during the winter months as the temperature tends to fluctuate between the cold of the outdoors and the warm indoors. In addition the dryness caused by heating also adds to the chances of the lips becoming damaged. These small cracks can increase in size and may eventually grow to become small cuts if left untreated. To avoid the initial formation of these cracks the best option is to apply lip balm, ideally before the damage begins to occur, but if not, as soon as possible afterward.

There are many lip balms available on the market, but for a number of reasons, it's nearly always better to make your own at home. One reason I suggest this is a better option is simply so you know exactly what has gone into your lip balm and, in turn, what you are exposing your body to. If you've read any of my other books you'll know by now that the products we use on our bodies don't simply sit on the surface of our skin, but they pass through our skin and are taken into our bodies where there is the potential for them to accumulate over time. When you make your own lip balms at home you are actively taking responsibility for what you allow onto your skin and therefore into your body. While the amount of chemical which passes to our bodies via a lip balm may be minimal as we only tend to use small amounts, the fact is that they can still play a part in the introduction of chemical toxins to the body. When we include other sources such as shampoos, deodorants and makeup, you can imagine how these harsh chemicals and preservatives can add up and potentially cause damage to the body's organs.

Lets take a closer look into some of the ingredients used in many store-bought lip balms, starting with menthol, camphor, and phenol. These ingredients are added for their cooling effects, but they can also dry out the skin on your lips, which ironically can mean more cracking and flaking. Alcohol is another common ingredient, usually listed as OL. This alcohol dries out quickly, and again can leave your lips dry and chapped. Lastly, they also use salicylic acid which is added to help peel off dry skin. Again, this harsh chemical can eventually lead to more chapping and flaking. The homemade lip balms in this book contain none of these harmful ingredients, meaning your lips will be spared the damaging side effects of store-bought lip balms mentioned above.

In addition, making your own lip balms at home is fun and many of the recipes in this book will allow you to create organic balms at a fraction of the price of the store-bought variety. Best of all, you get to customize your lip balm according to your preferences. You can choose which color, shimmer or scent you want to put on your lip balm or simply make a clear lip balm if you prefer. Once you get the hang of it, making your own lip balms at home is super easy and if you have extra they can stored in the fridge or given away as gifts for friends and family.

Technically, you only need two base ingredients to make a lip balm – beeswax and oil. You can choose from many different oils such as coconut oil, olive oil, almond oil, avocado oil, grapeseed oil and apricot kernel oil. From here it's basically a case of adding some essential oils and/or food grade coloring according to your preference. It really is as simple as that!

Let's take a look at some of the carrier oils that can be used when making lip balms at home and go into a little more detail on each.

Chapter 2

Carrier Oils & Butters Ideal For Lip Balms

A little later in this book, when you get to the recipes, you'll notice that each of the ingredients lists will include one or more carrier oil. They serve as the base oil of the lip balm and also play an important part in diluting the essential oils and fragrances so they can be applied on the skin.

Each of the carrier oils offers its own benefits and characteristics. Listed below are the carrier oils which are ideal for use in lip balms. Most are used in at lease one of the recipes in this book but a few are not. When you become a little more experienced with making lip balms feel free to try out new carrier oils to test their effects for yourself.

- **Almond Oil**- It is best to use the cold pressed/ unrefined version of this oil. The color of the oil is usually a very light gold or almost clear and the oil has a very slight, distinct nutty aroma. Almond Oil works great for all skin types and is suitable for sensitive skin. It can soothe and heal inflamed, dry skin leaving it soft and smooth.

- **Aloe Vera Oil** – This carrier oil is clear in color and odorless. It is great for lip balms because it works well for all skin types. It is also very hydrating, making it great for dry, flaky lips.

- **Apricot Kernel Oil** – This carrier oil is rich in linoleic and oleic acids, which are healthy fatty acids. It has a clear color with a tinge of yellow and a very faint aroma. It works well for all skin types and is easily absorbed by the skin so it does not feel greasy and moisturizers dry skin deeply.

- **Argan Oil**- This oil has an almost golden brown appearance and contains a high level of vitamin E and antioxidants. It has anti-inflammatory properties that help relieve inflamed, dry skin.

- **Avocado Oil** – It has a rich green color and a slightly fruity aroma. It is known for its healing and anti-wrinkle properties and is also antibacterial.

- **Blueberry Seed Oil** - This carrier oil is a rich green color with, perhaps unsurprisingly, a slight blueberry scent. It has very potent antioxidant properties and can help condition the skin. It is not overly-greasy, making it ideal for lip balms.

- **Brazil Nut Oil** – This oil has a clear yellow color with a hint of nutty aroma. It's a very rich carrier oil with 70% fat content. It also contains a significant level of selenium making it a great lubricant and skin conditioner.

- **Calendula Oil** – Widely used in skin care products such as creams, salves and balms due to its anti-inflammatory properties. It is very soothing to the skin and is great for repairing damaged tissues and promoting better blood circulation.

- **Camellia Oil** – This oil is yellow in color and comes from the seed of the camellia. It is composed of 80% Oleic Acid and is excellent in conditioning both the skin and hair.

- **Castor Oil** – Clear in color and easily combined with other oils. It has excellent lubricating properties and gives your lip balm a glossy look.

- **Chardonnay Grape Seed** – Has a slight green color with a lovely distinct aroma. It is easily absorbed by the skin so does not feel greasy.

- **Cherry Kernel Oil** – Has a light gold color with a hint of cherry scent. It conditions the skin while protecting it, leaving it smooth and soft.

- **Coconut Oil** – This carrier oil has a very long shelf life, lasting up to 4 years and can also help prevent other oils it is mixed with from going off, making it a superb natural preservative. It has a creamy, milky aroma that is distinct to coconuts as well as excellent conditioning properties that leave a protective layer on the skin.

- **Cranberry Seed Oil** – Used mainly due to its excellent emollient properties. It is also great for conditioning the skin and hair. It is golden-yellow to orange in color.

- **Hazelnut Oil** – This yellow carrier oil contains vitamins, minerals and protein. It is easily absorbed and helps keep the skin firm and elastic. It also helps tighten skin and promotes cell regeneration as well as stimulating blood circulation.

- **Hemp Seed Oil** – This oil has a slight nutty aroma and a rich, deep green color. It contains Vit A, Vit B1,Vit B2, Vit B3,Vit B6, Vit C,Vit D and Vit E. It effectively soothes and restores damaged and dry skin as well as increasing the skin's moisture retention. When used regularly, it can slow down the effects of aging and leave the skin soft, moisturized, and smooth.

- **Jojoba Oil** – This carrier oil is commonly used in body creams, salves and balms due to its long life. It can lasts up to 5 years and helps extend the life of other oils. It contains minerals and proteins and mimics collagen in its effects. It can also act as a sort of "second skin", protecting your own skin allowing it to breathe.

- **Kukui Nut Oil** – This oil is one of the lightest carrier oils. It penetrates into the skin deeply, preventing it from drying out without having a greasy feeling.

- **Mango Oil** – This oil is clear gold in color and is great for lip balms as it revitalizes and conditions the skin, keeping it smooth and flake-free.

- **Marula Oil** – High in anti-oxidants and oleic acid, this oil is very rich and is quickly absorbed by the skin, making it ideal for lip balms as well as other skin care products.

- **Meadowfoam Oil** – This oil also has a long shelf life – up to 5 years. It is very stable oil and also a wonderful lubricant. It is able to condition the skin and lock in moisture.

- **Olive Oil** – Rich in vitamins, minerals, proteins and fatty acids. Aside from its anti-oxidant properties, it cleanses, conditions, and softens the skin. It is also easily absorbed by the skin.

- **Peach Kernel Oil** – Used mainly due to it conditioning properties. It is also non-greasy and deep-penetrating.

- **Pecan Nut Oil** – A very rich oil but highly nourishing for the skin. It heals dry, damaged skin while keeping it conditioned.

- **Plum Kernel Oil** – It's slightly fruity aroma makes it a great addition to lip balm recipes. It is a rich and exotic oil that deeply penetrates the skin without feeling greasy. It has a high fatty-acid content and excellent anti-oxidant properties.

- **Pomegranate Seed Oil** – This oil is rich in fiber and lipids. It is antibacterial and it also nourishes and conditions the skin. It smoothens fine lines and wrinkles, restores the skin's Ph balance and keeps the skin smooth and well-nourished.

- **Poppy Seed Oil** – Contains minerals, proteins, and linoleic acids. It conditions the skin and keeps it smooth and moisturized.

- **Rice Bran Oil** – This carrier oil is high in fatty acids and ferulic acids. It conditions the skin and keeps it soft.

- **Rose Hip Seed Oil** – Has a very high fatty acid content and can have remarkable effects on dry, damaged and mature skin.

- **Safflower Oil** – Has a shelf life of two years and is a very light yellow in color. Has excellent conditioning properties!

- **Shea Oil** – This oil comes from the seed of the Karite Tree and is usually yellow or gold in appearance. It has anti-inflammatory properties and feels great when applied to the skin.

- **Strawberry Seed Oil** – This is a rich carrier oil that has a light yellow color. It is deep penetrating and is absorbed easily by the body. It also protects and nourishes the skin and has anti-aging properties.

- **Sunflower Oil** – This carrier oil is very cost-effective. It has skin conditioning properties and keeps the skin smooth.

- **Walnut Oil** – An extremely effective moisturizer for dry and damaged skin.

- **Watermelon Seed Oil** – High in Omega 6 and 9 fatty acids. It is transdermal and it has fantastic healing properties.

- **Wheat Germ Oil**- This oil comes from the wheat kernel and is considered a valuable addition to any skin care product. It has high levels of vitamin E and deeply nourishes the skin.

If you're looking to experiment and try your own recipes, a basic rule is to mix 1 part oil, 1 part butter, and 1 part beeswax. For example you could mix 1-tablespoon of walnut oil with a tablespoon of Shea butter and a tablespoon of beeswax. As you become accustomed to the process you can adjust the combinations slightly to suit your own preferences. If you prefer a firmer lip balm simply add one more tablespoon of beeswax. Beeswax comes in either pastilles or blocks. If you have it in block-form, you will have to shave it to get an accurate measurement. This will also speed up the melting time.

If you want to add fragrance to your lip balms, start by adding 10 drops. Make sure to check with the manufacturer if the product is food grade. This is important as you are using the product on your lips and there is a good chance that you will ingest a small amount of it.

For the butters, there are several that you can choose from.

- **Shea Butter** – Commonly used for skin care products because it's not overly greasy and is virtually odorless. It has anti-inflammatory and antioxidant properties and is an excellent moisturizer which helps reduce the appearance of wrinkles and stretch marks. It is also known to relieve eczema and psoriasis.

- **Mango Butter** – Works wonders on the skin! It is rich in fiber, vitamin A, vitamin C and potassium.

- **Cocoa Butter** – An excellent moisturizer, cocoa butter boosts elastin and collagen production as well as helping to minimize the appearance of stretch marks and scars. Aside from smelling really good, it also relieves dermatitis flare-ups and eczema.

- **Coconut Cream** – Coconut has excellent antibacterial, antiviral and anti-inflammatory properties. It also has great healing properties and is excellent in repairing damaged tissues. And of course, it's a fantastic moisturizer and wrinkle-buster!

When you start experimenting with your own recipes, the oil or butter you choose for your lip balm will depend on the properties you'd like it to have. Keep in mind that there some of the oils and butters are very expensive while others are much cheaper.

The shelf life of your lip balms depends on how you store them. If unused, you can keep them in the fridge for at least a few months. Just be sure to check the lip balm smells fresh and the consistency hasn't altered dramatically since you made it, and the balm should be good to use.

There are times, especially during summer, when the oils used in the balm become softer. If this happens, just place the lip balm in the fridge for a few hours to set. Also, some oils become rancid more quickly than others. You can add a few drops of vitamin E into your recipe to make the balm last longer as it acts as a natural preservative and should keep your lip balm fresh for up to a year.

Chapter 3

Insider Tips On Creating Your Own Lip Balms

It doesn't matter where you got your inspiration from, the important thing is that you've taken that first step to using much healthier, non-harmful lip balms. Making your own lip balms will be a lot of fun, but there are some things you should be aware of before you begin. So before you grab that mixing bowl, here are a few insider tips to get you off to a good start and help you avoid any problems further down the road.

Prep your workspace

The first thing you need to do before you get started on making your lip balms is to prep your workspace. Making your own lip balms at home can get quite messy, so make sure that you have prepared a dedicated space for it which will be easy to clean up when you've finished. Working in the kitchen is perfectly fine, but if you're going to turn it into a habit, you might want to look around your home for a small area you can dedicate to lip balm creation, space permitting of course.

Source your ingredients from a reliable supplier

Most of the ingredients needed to make your own homemade lip balm can easily be bought locally.

However, if you're looking for an ingredient that can't be easily purchased in your area, you can always find a reliable supplier online with a little searching. When sourcing ingredients, make sure to choose a supplier that is known first and foremost for their quality, and not just the quantity of product they are offering. Don't be fooled by a cheap price tag if you're not sure about the quality of the product. Think of these ingredients as you would food; they will be entering your body through your skin, so chose the best you can find or that you can afford.

Be aware of your allergies

Just because an ingredient is considered all-natural or organic doesn't mean that it's guaranteed to be 100% safe for you. It may work wonders for others, but there is the odd chance that for you it could cause an allergic reaction. So before you get started on any homemade lip balms, make sure that the ingredients you're going to use are safe for you. Try to figure out which (if any) of the ingredients may cause skin irritation. If you're going to work with an unfamiliar ingredient, test it first on your wrist to see if it causes a negative reaction. This way, you don't end up harming your skin in your quest for healthier lip balm alternatives.

Start with small batches

Since your homemade lip balm doesn't contain any chemical ingredients designed to prolong its lifespan, it's best to only make small batches at a time. Most of the recipes in this book will last for a matter of weeks, depending on the product. Therefore, it's highly recommended that you don't make too much at one time. However, as making fresh batches is quick, easy and fun, creating more is unlikely to be a major inconvenience.

Always store homemade lip balm in appropriate containers

Once you've made a fresh batch of DIY lip balm, it's critical that you store it in an appropriate container. As I mentioned above, your homemade lip balm won't contain any chemical preservatives to prevent bacterial growth, so always make it a point to use sterile containers. Look for containers with airtight lids so your product won't be exposed to air, humidity, germs, and bacteria. Although not essential, glass containers are a good option as glass is inert, meaning no chemicals will be able to leach into your lip balm.

Don't get too hung up on following the recipes to the letter

The amounts of the ingredients you'll need may seem a little vague (for example "1/8 cup" or "¼ teaspoon") but don't get too hung up on being exact; just follow the instructions as best you can to begin with. Making your own lip balms is a lot like cooking; over time you'll get used to the recipes and will be able to adjust them to suit your own needs and preferences.

Now that you're well prepared, let's get started on the recipes! Ive broken the recipes down into chapters based on type. Good luck!

Chapter 4

Fruity Lip Balm Recipes

Fruity lip balms are especially great for summer. The sweet, fruity aromas of these lip balms will help keep you feeling refreshed and invigorated. So, if you want fantastically fruity smelling, smooth, supple lips, apply one of these amazing fruity lip balms. In addition, believe it or not, since they are all-natural you can even use a little of these lip balms as a makeshift moisturizer if you run out!

1. Citrus Burst

A mixture of orange, tangerine and grapefruit essential oils, this lip balm is simply bursting with sweet, citrus aroma! Great for improving your energy levels as well as keeping your lips moisturized throughout the day.

Ingredients:

- 3 teaspoons beeswax (pellets or grated)

- 5 teaspoons jojoba oil

- 3 drops orange essential oil

- 3 drops tangerine essential oil

- 2 drops grapefruit essential oil

- 1 teaspoon honey

Instructions:

1. In a double boiler*, melt the beeswax together with the jojoba oil. Stir to combine.

2. Remove from heat. Stir in the honey thoroughly being sure to avoid clumping. Add in the essential oils and mix thoroughly until combined.

3. Pour the mixture into individual containers. Do not cap the containers but cover loosely with a cloth or tea towel to stop any dust or other particles from settling on the lip balms. Allow to settle and cool for about an hour or until you're sure the lip balm has hardened. Cap the containers. Store extra lip balms in the refrigerator to prolong their usefulness. In the

fridge these lip balms should last from a few months to a year.

*If you do not have a double boiler, you can use a glass bowl placed in a pot of simmering water instead.

2. Strawberry Glitter Lip Balm

This lip balm gives off a sweet, fruity scent and flavor that's both invigorating and uplifting. If you decide to add the natural food coloring it's pinkish appearance will also give your lips that cutesy, girly look!

Ingredients:

- 4 tablespoons sunflower oil

- 2 tablespoons beeswax (pellets or grated)

- 6 drops strawberry essential oil

- 2 drops red liquid food coloring (optional - leave out for a colorless lip balm)

Instructions:

1. In a glass jug, mix together the beeswax and the sunflower oil.

2. Melt in the microwave being sure not to boil. When completely melted, remove the jug from the microwave and stir with a metal spoon until the ingredients are combined.

3. Add the 2 drops of red liquid food coloring and mix well until the color is even. Add extra drops of coloring for a darker lip gloss.

4. Pour the mixture into individual containers. Do not cap the containers but cover loosely with a cloth or tea towel to stop any dust or other particles from settling on the lip balms. Allow to settle and cool for about an hour or until you're sure the lip balm has hardened. Cap the

containers. Store extra lip balms in the refrigerator to prolong their usefulness. In the fridge these lip balms should last from a few months to a year.

3. Summer Fresh Lip Balm

This lip balm recipe contains coconut oil, which acts as a fantastic deep moisturizer, leaving your lips smooth and silky-soft.

Ingredients:

- 1 tablespoon virgin coconut oil

- 1 tablespoon beeswax (pellets or grated)

- 1 teaspoon honey

- 2 capsules vitamin E*

- 3 drops mandarin essential oil

- 3 drops lemon essential oil

- 2 drops spearmint essential oil

Instructions:

1. Melt the beeswax in a double boiler**. When approximately half of the beeswax has melted, add in the coconut oil and stir.

2. Continue to heat and stir the mixture until the beeswax has completely melted and the two ingredients are thoroughly combined. At this point remove from the heat.

3. Stir in the honey until well combined and there are no clumps in the mixture. Add the essential oils and stir again briefly.

4. Carefully, prick the vitamin E capsules with a pin and squeeze the contents into the mixture. Stir once again.

5. Pour the mixture into individual containers. Do not cap the containers but cover loosely with a cloth or tea towel to stop any dust or other particles from settling on the lip balms. Allow to settle and cool for about an hour or until you're sure the lip balm has hardened. Cap the containers. Store extra lip balms in the refrigerator to prolong their usefulness. In the fridge these lip balms should last from a few months to a year.

*As well as helping keep your skin in good condition, vitamin E acts as a natural preservative, which can help prolong the life of your lip balm for to up to a year!

**If you do not have a double boiler, you can use a glass bowl placed in a pot of simmering water instead.

4. Citrus Mint Lip Balm

On hot summer days, it's important to keep our lips well moisturized in order to prevent chapping and flaking. As well as helping to lock in moisture and keep lips hydrated for longer, the peppermint essential oil in this lip balm helps keep lips feeling fresh and cool!

Ingredients:

- 2 tablespoons beeswax (pellets or grated)

- 4 tablespoons sunflower oil

- 4 drops peppermint essential oil

- 3 drops tangerine essential oil

- 2 drops lemon essential oil

Instructions:

1. In a glass jug, combine the beeswax and the sunflower oil.

2. Heat in the microwave until the beeswax is completely melted. Be sure not to boil the mixture.

3. Remove from the microwave and stir thoroughly with a metal spoon. Add the essential oils and stir again until well combined.

4. Pour the mixture into individual containers. Do not cap the containers but cover loosely with a cloth or tea towel to stop any dust or other particles from settling on the lip balms. Allow to settle and cool for about an hour or until you're sure the lip balm has hardened. Cap the containers. Store extra lip balms in the

refrigerator to prolong their usefulness. In the fridge these lip balms should last from a few months to a year.

5. Lemon Vanilla Lip Balm

If you are looking for a sweet, citrusy lip balm, this one is for you! Since it's made with coconut oil, it's super-hydrating and a little bit of this lip balm goes a really long way!

Ingredients:

- 1 tablespoon Shea butter

- 1 tablespoon beeswax (pellets or grated)

- 2 tablespoons coconut oil

- 3 drops lemon essential oil

- 2 drops vanilla essential oil

- Natural food coloring of your choice (optional - leave out for a colorless lip balm)

Instructions:

1. Place the Shea butter, beeswax, and coconut oil into a glass jar or large glass bowl. Place the glass jar/bowl into a pot of simmering water. Mix until the ingredients are melted. Be careful not to allow the water to go into the mixture.

2. Remove from the heat and add the essential oils.

3. Add the coloring (if you've chosen to use it) and mix in until the color is even.

4. Pour the mixture into individual containers. Do not cap the containers but cover loosely with a cloth or tea towel to stop any dust or other particles from settling on the lip balms. Allow to

settle and cool for about an hour or until you're sure the lip balm has hardened. Cap the containers. Store extra lip balms in the refrigerator to prolong their usefulness. In the fridge these lip balms should last from a few months to a year.

6. Minty Lemon Blend

The zesty, citrus scent of lemon is invigorating and refreshing. Blended with jojoba oil, this lip balm effectively moisturizes the lips, coating them with a nourishing, protective layer which prevents drying.

Ingredients:

- 2 tablespoons beeswax (pellets or grated)

- 1 tablespoon jojoba oil

- 1 tablespoon Shea butter

- 2 vitamin E capsules

- 15 drops lemon essential oil

- 10 drops eucalyptus essential oil

Instructions:

1. Place the beeswax, jojoba oil and Shea butter in a double boiler or glass container placed in a pot of simmering water. Heat gently and stir until the beeswax is melted and the ingredients are thoroughly combined.

2. Carefully, prick the vitamin E capsules with a pin and squeeze the contents into the mixture. Add the essential oils and mix the ingredients together. Remove from the heat and stir again.

3. Pour the mixture into individual containers. Do not cap the containers but cover loosely with a cloth or tea towel to stop any dust or other particles from settling on the lip balms. Allow to settle and cool for about an hour or until you're

sure the lip balm has hardened. Cap the containers. Store extra lip balms in the refrigerator to prolong their usefulness. In the fridge these lip balms should last from a few months to a year.

Chapter 5

Floral Lip Balm Recipes

These next lip balms have wonderfully relaxing floral fragrances that will help uplift your mood and destress your mind and body.

The flowery aroma of these floral lip balms, blended with citrus, vanilla, or minty essences offers a fantastically different aroma.

7. Sweet Floral Lip Balm

This lip balm contains jasmine essential oil which gives it a sweet, floral scent, making it great for enhancing your mood and relaxing your mind.

Ingredients:

- 1 tablespoon beeswax (pellets or grated)

- 2 tablespoons mango butter

- 2 tablespoons coconut oil

- 15 drops jasmine essential oil

- 5 drops lavender essential oil

Instructions:

1. Gently simmer about ½ cup of water in a small pot.

2. Place the beeswax, mango butter and coconut oil in a glass jar or small bowl. Gently place this jar into the pot of simmering water. Be careful not to get any water into the jar.

3. Mix until all the ingredients are well-combined.

4. Turn off the heat and let the jar sit in the pot. Stir in the essential oils.

5. Pour the mixture into individual containers. Do not cap the containers but cover loosely with a cloth or tea towel to stop any dust or other particles from settling on the lip balms. Allow to settle and cool for about an hour or until you're sure the lip balm has hardened. Cap the containers. Store extra lip balms in the

refrigerator to prolong their usefulness. In the fridge these lip balms should last from a few months to a year.

8. Cool Flower

This lip balm gives you the sweet, floral aroma of lavender and geranium with a slight kick of peppermint, and will help give you a boost on a busy day.

Ingredients:

- 2 tablespoons beeswax (pellets or grated)

- 2 tablespoons coconut oil

- 2 tablespoons Shea butter

- 10 drops lavender essential oil

- 10 drops geranium essential oil

- 5 drops peppermint essential oil

- 1 vitamin E capsule

Instructions:

1. If you have a double boiler, you may use it. If not, fill a pot with a few inches of water and simmer on medium heat. Place a glass jar in the simmering water. Be careful not to get any water in the glass jar.

2. Place beeswax, coconut oil and Shea butter in the glass jar. Mix until melted. Remove from heat.

3. Carefully prick the vitamin E capsule with a pin and squeeze the contents into the mixture. Also add the essential oil. Mix thoroughly.

4. Pour the mixture into individual containers. Do not cap the containers but cover loosely with a cloth or tea towel to stop any dust or other

particles from settling on the lip balms. Allow to settle and cool for about an hour or until you're sure the lip balm has hardened. Cap the containers. Store extra lip balms in the refrigerator to prolong their usefulness. In the fridge these lip balms should last from a few months to a year.

9. Pretty In Pink Lip Balm

If you're after supple, natural-looking lips, you may want to try this lip balm. It contains coral pink mica for coloring, so it also gives your lips a slight shimmer.

Ingredients:

- 1 tablespoon Shea butter

- 1 tablespoon mango butter

- 1 tablespoon olive oil

- 1 tablespoon beeswax (pellets or grated)

- 1/8 teaspoon coral pink mica (optional - leave out for a colorless lip balm)

- 5 drops rose essential oil

- 5 drops geranium essential oil

- 5 drops jasmine essential oil

Instructions:

1. In a pot, melt Shea butter, mango butter, and beeswax pastilles over medium heat. Stir in olive oil.

2. Turn off heat. Add essential oils. Mix thoroughly.

3. Add the mica and mix thoroughly until color is even. Add more if you want a darker color.

4. Pour the mixture into individual containers. Do not cap the containers but cover loosely with a cloth or tea towel to stop any dust or other particles from settling on the lip balms. Allow to settle and cool for about an hour or until you're sure the lip balm has hardened. Cap the containers. Store extra lip balms in the refrigerator to prolong their usefulness. In the fridge these lip balms should last from a few months to a year.

10. Luscious Red Floral Lip Balm

When you are going out on a date and you don't feel like wearing lipstick, this lip balm is a great alternative. It gives your lips a sexy, subtle red color while keeping your lips moisturized, while exuding a sensual floral scent.

Ingredients:

- 2 tablespoons beeswax (pellets or grated)

- 1 tablespoon Shea butter

- 1 tablespoon coconut oil

- ½ teaspoon red mica (optional - leave out for a colorless lip balm)

- 10 drops rose essential oil

- 5 drops vanilla essential oil

- 5 drops tea tree oil

Instructions:

1. Combine beeswax, Shea butter, and coconut oil in a glass jar or bowl.

2. Pour a few inches of water in a saucepan and simmer over medium heat. Do not boil. Place the glass jar or bowl in the saucepan with the simmering water.

3. Mix until the oil and butter are completely blended. Stir in the essential oils.

4. Add the mica until you reach the desired color. Mix thoroughly until the color is evenly distributed through the mixture.

5. Pour the mixture into individual containers. Do not cap the containers but cover loosely with a cloth or tea towel to stop any dust or other particles from settling on the lip balms. Allow to settle and cool for about an hour or until you're sure the lip balm has hardened. Cap the containers. Store extra lip balms in the refrigerator to prolong their usefulness. In the fridge these lip balms should last from a few months to a year.

11. Rosy Sensation Lip Balm

Made from all-natural ingredients, this lip balm is fantastic for your lips. It's made from real rose petals giving it a sensual scent and alkanet root powder which gives it its natural red color. Organic lip balm has never been this hydrating or sensual!

Ingredients:

Lip Balm

- 1 tablespoon Shea butter

- 1 tablespoon beeswax (pellets or grated)

- 3 tablespoons rose infused oil

- ½ tablespoon castor oil

- Powdered alkanet root

- 15 drops peppermint essential oil

Rose Infused Oil

- Dried rose petals

- Sunflower oil

- Glass jar (with wide mouth)

Instructions:

1. For the rose infused oil: Fill ¾ of the glass jar with dried rose petals. Pour the sunflower oil into the jar until all the rose petals are completely covered.

2. There are two ways to infuse the oil. One way is to cover the mouth of the glass jar with a few layers of cheesecloth. Tie the rim with rubber band to secure the cheesecloth. Place the glass jar in a

cool, dry place, away from direct sunlight for 3 to 4 weeks.

3. For a faster infusion, place the glass jar of rose petals with oil in a pot filled with a few inches of water. Turn on heat on low. Simmer gently for two hours making sure to replace the water if it boils off.

4. When the infusion process is complete, strain the oil and discard the rose petals. The rose infused oil is now ready to be used to make your lip balm!

5. For the lip balm: Pour a teaspoon of rose infused oil into a bowl. Stir in the alkanet powder, a little at a time until you form a red paste. This will serve as your natural lip balm colorant.

6. In a deep glass bowl, place the Shea butter, castor oil, beeswax and the remaining rose infused oil.

Place in a pot of simmering water until all ingredients have melted.

7. Add the paste you made with the alkanet root powder a little at a time until the desired color is achieved. Remove from heat. Add the essential oil and mix well.

8. Pour the mixture into individual containers. Do not cap the containers but cover loosely with a cloth or tea towel to stop any dust or other particles from settling on the lip balms. Allow to settle and cool for about an hour or until you're sure the lip balm has hardened. Cap the containers. Store extra lip balms in the refrigerator to prolong their usefulness. In the fridge these lip balms should last from a few months to a year.

Chapter 6

Cool Mint Lip Balm Recipes

It's always nice to feel that cooling effect on your lips especially during hot and humid days. These cool mint lip balm recipes will give you that fresh, cool feeling while keeping your lips supple and looking great.

These lip balms are great during summer for that refreshing, cool feeling. They can also help open a clogged nose and sinuses so they can also be great if you have a cold or flu.

12. Relaxing Eucalyptus Lip Balm

Eucalyptus is known for its decongestant properties that are very handy when you are suffering from a cold or have a clogged nose. With its refreshing and relaxing aroma, this lip balm is sure to give you a boost while leaving you with lovely soft, lips.

Ingredients:

- 1 tablespoon beeswax (pellets or grated)

- 1 tablespoon sweet almond oil

- 1 tablespoon coconut oil

- 5 drops eucalyptus essential oil

Instructions:

1. Simmer water in a double boiler. Melt together the coconut oil, almond oil and beeswax.

2. Remove from heat and stir in the essential oil. Mix thoroughly until all   of the ingredients are combined.

3. Pour the mixture into individual containers. Do not cap the containers but cover loosely with a cloth or tea towel to stop any dust or other particles from settling on the lip balms. Allow to settle and cool for about an hour or until you're sure the lip balm has hardened. Cap the containers. Store extra lip balms in the refrigerator to prolong their usefulness. In the fridge these lip balms should last from a few months to a year.

13. Cooling Peppermint Lip Balm

Peppermint has a cooling effect that effectively refreshes not only your lips but also your mind and body. It can also help reduce itchiness and irritation so this lip balm is particularly useful of you're suffering from damaged or sensitive lips.

Ingredients:

- 1 tablespoon virgin coconut oil

- 1 teaspoon beeswax (pellets or grated)

- 2 capsules of vitamin E

- 25 drops peppermint essential oil

Instructions:

1. Pour a few inches of water in a pot and simmer over medium heat. Make sure you don't boil the water.

2. Place the coconut oil and beeswax in a glass bowl or container. Carefully, prick the vitamin E capsules with a pin and squeeze the contents into the container. Put the glass container in the pot of simmering water. Mix until the oils liquify and the ingredients are thoroughly combined.

3. Remove from the heat and immediately add the essential oil. Mix again.

4. Pour the mixture into individual containers. Do not cap the containers but cover loosely with a cloth or tea towel to stop any dust or other

particles from settling on the lip balms. Allow to settle and cool for about an hour or until you're sure the lip balm has hardened. Cap the containers. Store extra lip balms in the refrigerator to prolong their usefulness. In the fridge these lip balms should last from a few months to a year.

14. Minty Fresh Lip Balm

If you are looking for something for your lips that is sweet yet cool and minty, this lip balm recipe will be perfect with it's mixture of peppermint, eucalyptus and tea tree essential oils with a hint of chamomile and orange & tangerine.

Ingredients:

- 2 tablespoons beeswax (pellets or grated)

- 1 tablespoon mango butter

- 1 tablespoon cocoa butter

- 1 tablespoon coconut oil

- 15 drops peppermint essential oil

- 10 drops eucalyptus essential oil

- 5 drops tea tree oil

- 3 drops orange essential oil

- 2 drops tangerine essential oil

Instructions:

1. Place a few inches of water in a pot. Simmer over medium heat but do not boil. Feel free to use a double boiler if you have one.

2. Put the beeswax, mango butter, cocoa butter and coconut oil in a glass bowl or glass jar. Mix until all the ingredients are melted and liquid in consistency.

3. Add the essential oils, remove from the heat and continue stirring.

4. Pour the mixture into individual containers. Do not cap the containers but cover loosely with a cloth or tea towel to stop any dust or other particles from settling on the lip balms. Allow to settle and cool for about an hour or until you're sure the lip balm has hardened. Cap the containers. Store extra lip balms in the refrigerator to prolong their usefulness. In the fridge these lip balms should last from a few months to a year.

15. Minty Spice Lip Balm

This lip balm is not only refreshing; it also has a tinge of spiciness to add an extra kick to the taste of this lip balm!

Ingredients:

- 1 tablespoon beeswax (pellets or grated)

- 1 tablespoon sweet almond oil

- 1 tablespoon peach kernel oil

- 1 capsule vitamin E

- 10 drops peppermint essential oil

- 5 drops eucalyptus essential oil

- 6 drops ginger essential oil

- 4 drops ylang-ylang essential oil

Instructions:

1. Put the beeswax, almond oil and peach kernel oil into a glass bowl or glass jar. Carefully, prick the vitamin E capsule with a pin and squeeze the contents into the bowl/jar. Place this bowl or jar into a pot filled with a few inches of simmering water and melt the beeswax.

2. Mix the ingredients in the jar together thoroughly. Turn off heat but do not remove the jar from the pot.

3. Stir in the essential oils. Remove from the hot water and keep stirring to fully incorporate all ingredients.

4. Pour the mixture into individual containers. Do not cap the containers but cover loosely with a cloth or tea towel to stop any dust or other particles from settling on the lip balms. Allow to settle and cool for about an hour or until you're sure the lip balm has hardened. Cap the containers. Store extra lip balms in the refrigerator to prolong their usefulness. In the fridge these lip balms should last from a few months to a year.

16. Fruit Mint Lip Balm

This fruity and minty lip balm cools and deeply moisturizes your lips. It also has a fantastically fresh, fruity, citrus aroma with an air of sweetness!

Ingredients:

- 2 tablespoons beeswax (pellets or grated)

- 1 tablespoon coconut oil

- 1 tablespoon hazelnut oil

- 1 tablespoon strawberry seed oil

- 1 capsule vitamin E

- 10 drops peppermint essential oil

- 10 drops star anise essential oil

- 5 drops lemon essential oil

Instructions:

1. Simmer ½ cup of water in a pot over medium heat.

2. Place the beeswax, coconut oil, hazelnut oil, and strawberry seed oil in a glass jar or glass bowl. Carefully, prick the vitamin E capsule with a pin and squeeze the contents into the mixture.

3. Put the jar in the pot of simmering water. Reduce the heat to the lowest setting. Mix the oils until all the ingredients have melted. Turn off the heat but leave the jar in the pot.

4. Stir in all the essential oil. Remove from pot and stir once more.

5. Pour the mixture into individual containers. Do not cap the containers but cover loosely with a cloth or tea towel to stop any dust or other particles from settling on the lip balms. Allow to settle and cool for about an hour or until you're sure the lip balm has hardened. Cap the containers. Store extra lip balms in the refrigerator to prolong their usefulness. In the fridge these lip balms should last from a few months to a year.

Chapter 7

Vanilla Lip Balm Recipes

Vanilla has always been a favorite for so many because of it's wonderful aroma. What's more, these vanilla-based lip balm recipes are not only soothing and hydrating for your lips; you can even use them as makeshift moisturizers on other parts of your body which may need deep moisturizing, such as your elbows, knees, and feet!

17. Happy Lips Lip Balm

This lip balm consists of a combination of a number of wonderful ingredients which, when combined, give the most magnificent aroma!

Ingredients:

- 1 tablespoon walnut oil

- 1 tablespoon sunflower oil

- 1 tablespoon safflower oil

- 2 tablespoons beeswax (pellets or grated)

- 1 teaspoon honey

- 10 drops vanilla essential oil

- 10 drops strawberry essential oil

- 5 drops lemon essential oil

- 5 drops tangerine essential oil

Instructions:

1. In a double boiler or a glass bowl placed in a pot of simmering water, heat the carrier oils (walnut, sunflower, and safflower) and the beeswax.

2. When completely melted, turn off the heat but do not remove the jar from the pot of simmering water or double boiler. Mix in the honey thoroughly until it is well incorporated with the oils and beeswax.

3. Add the essential oils (vanilla, strawberry, lemon and tangerine) and stir until well-

blended. Remove from the pot of hot water and stir once more.

4. Pour the mixture into individual containers. Do not cap the containers but cover loosely with a cloth or tea towel to stop any dust or other particles from settling on the lip balms. Allow to settle and cool for about an hour or until you're sure the lip balm has hardened. Cap the containers. Store extra lip balms in the refrigerator to prolong their usefulness. In the fridge these lip balms should last from a few months to a year.

18. Sweet Sensation Lip Balm

This lip balm has a highly intoxicating sweet smell that can be near to addicting. The oils used are high hydrating and penetrate the skin deeply so your lips stay soft longer.

Ingredients:

- 1 tablespoon plum kernel oil

- 1 tablespoon strawberry seed oil

- 1 tablespoon virgin coconut oil

- 2 tablespoons beeswax (pellets or grated)

- 10 drops vanilla essential oil

- 10 drops geranium essential oil

- 5 drops strawberry essential oil

Instructions:

1. In a pot, melt the beeswax, coconut oil, strawberry seed oil and plum kernel oil over the lowest heat possible.

2. When completely melted, stir in the essential oils.

3. Turn off the heat and stir once more.

4. Pour the mixture into individual containers. Do not cap the containers but cover loosely with a cloth or tea towel to stop any dust or other particles from settling on the lip balms. Allow to settle and cool for about an hour or until you're sure the lip balm has hardened. Cap the containers. Store extra lip balms in the

refrigerator to prolong their usefulness. In the fridge these lip balms should last from a few months to a year.

19. Choco Vanilla Lip Balm

The sweet blend of chocolate and vanilla produces a lip-balm which is as good as it sounds! Not only does it taste amazing, the cocoa butter in the recipe will leave your lips feeling super-soft and smooth.

Ingredients:

- 1 tablespoon cocoa butter

- 1 tablespoon aloe vera oil

- 1 tablespoon almond oil

- 2 tablespoons beeswax (pellets or grated)

- 1 teaspoon pure vanilla extract

- 5 drops star anise essential oil

Instructions:

1. Melt the carrier oils and beeswax in a double boiler or in a glass container placed in a pot of simmering water.

2. When melted, add the vanilla extract and essential oil.

3. Remove from the heat and mix thoroughly.

4. Pour the mixture into individual containers. Do not cap the containers but cover loosely with a cloth or tea towel to stop any dust or other particles from settling on the lip balms. Allow to settle and cool for about an hour or until you're sure the lip balm has hardened. Cap the containers. Store extra lip balms in the refrigerator to prolong their usefulness. In the

fridge these lip balms should last from a few

months to a year.

20. Vanilla and Herbs Lip Balm

The chamomile, basil and lavender in this recipe produce a sweet, almost minty aroma when mixed together. When you add vanilla to the mix it infuses this wonderful aroma with a touch of a sweet floral scent.

Ingredients:

- 1 tablespoon mango butter

- 1 tablespoon sweet almond oil

- 1 tablespoon virgin coconut oil

- 2 tablespoons beeswax (pellets or grated)

- 1 teaspoon pure vanilla extract

- 10 drops chamomile essential oil

- 10 drops lavender essential oil

- 5 drops basil essential oil

Instructions:

1. Melt the mango butter, almond oil, coconut oil and beeswax in a double boiler or a small pot or jar placed in a pan of gently simmering water.

2. Stir in the vanilla extract and mix thoroughly.

3. Add in the essential oils and stir until the ingredients are well blended. Remove from the heat and stir once again.

4. Pour the mixture into individual containers. Do not cap the containers but cover loosely with a cloth or tea towel to stop any dust or other particles from settling on the lip balms. Allow to settle and cool for about an hour or until you're sure the lip balm has hardened. Cap the containers. Store extra lip balms in the refrigerator to prolong their usefulness. In the fridge these lip balms should last from a few months to a year.

21. Floral Honey Vanilla Lip Balm

Intense floral aromas with a blend of honey and vanilla; this deeply nourishing lip balm should leave you feeling uplifted in no time!

Ingredients:

- 2 tablespoons beeswax (pellets or grated)

- 1 tablespoon calendula oil

- 1 tablespoon camellia oil

- 1 tablespoon cocoa butter

- 1 tablespoon coconut cream

- 15 drops lavender essential oil

- 10 drops jasmine essential oil

- 1 teaspoon pure vanilla extract

- 1 teaspoon raw honey

Instructions:

1. Feel free to use a double boiler if you have one. Alternatively you can place the beeswax, calendula oil, camellia oil, cocoa butter and coconut cream into a glass container. Simmer ½ cup of water in a pot over medium heat and place the jar inside. Do not boil, just simmer.

2. Melt the oils and stir in the vanilla extract. Slowly add in the honey while stirring. Mix thoroughly and make sure the honey is well incorporated with the other ingredients. Turn off the heat but leave the jar in the pot.

3. Stir in the essential oils. Remove from the heat and give the mixture a few more swirls.

4. Pour the mixture into individual containers. Do not cap the containers but cover loosely with a cloth or tea towel to stop any dust or other particles from settling on the lip balms. Allow to settle and cool for about an hour or until you're sure the lip balm has hardened. Cap the containers. Store extra lip balms in the refrigerator to prolong their usefulness. In the fridge these lip balms should last from a few months to a year.

22. Rose Vanilla Lip Balm

The floral fresh aroma of rose combined with the sweet scent of vanilla creates a truly amazing lip balm that is especially suitable for any romantic occasions!

Ingredients:

- 2 tablespoons beeswax (pellets or grated)

- 1 tablespoon almond oil

- 1 tablespoon apricot kernel oil

- 1 tablespoon Shea butter

- 1 teaspoon pure vanilla extract

- 20 drops rose essential oil

Instructions:

1. Melt the beeswax, almond oil, apricot kernel oil and Shea butter in a glass container placed inside a pot with a few inches of simmering (not boiling) water.

2. As soon as the carrier oils and beeswax are melted, stir in the vanilla extract.

3. Add the essential oils and stir in. Remove from heat and mix once more.

4. Pour the mixture into individual containers. Do not cap the containers but cover loosely with a cloth or tea towel to stop any dust or other particles from settling on the lip balms. Allow to settle and cool for about an hour or until you're sure the lip balm has hardened. Cap the

containers. Store extra lip balms in the refrigerator to prolong their usefulness. In the fridge these lip balms should last from a few months to a year.

<u>Conclusion</u>

I hope you enjoyed this book and were able to learn a lot about the benefits of making your own homemade lip balms. What's more, I hope you will actually try some of these recipes for yourself and that you experience the benefits of using these natural, healthy alternatives!

A message from the author, Jane Aniston

Finally, if you enjoyed this book, **please** take the time to post a review on Amazon. It will only take a couple of minutes and I'd be extremely grateful for your support.

Jane Aniston

FREE BONUS!: Preview Of "Homemade Makeup - A Complete Beginner's Guide to Natural DIY Cosmetics You Can Make Today" - Includes 28 Organic Makeup Recipes!'

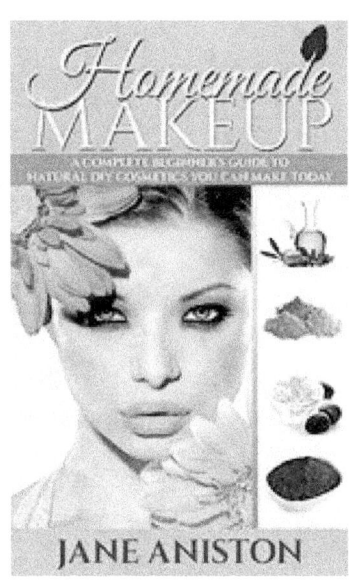

If you enjoyed this book, I have a little bonus for you; a preview of one of my other books "Homemade Makeup - A Complete Beginner's Guide to Natural DIY Cosmetics You Can Make Today", which exposes the secrets of the hidden toxins lurking in your store-bought cosmetics! This book also includes 28 simple and enjoyable organic makeup recipes that you can make at home today. Give yourself a glamorous look without exposing yourself to potentially harmful chemical nasties! Enjoy!

Chapter 1: Why you should stop using store-bought makeup and start making your own at home!

Makeup is something most women simply can't live without. Some women, in their search for beauty, have even gone as far getting permanent cosmetics tattooed on their faces (permanent eyebrows, for example). Personally, I see nothing wrong with wanting to look your best, but at the end of the day, one question we need to ask ourselves is: "What exactly are the ingredients in my beauty products?"

With almost all cosmetics containing numerous chemical ingredients, it can be a bit unsettling to think about the potential long-term effects these ingredients could be having on our bodies. Behind the glamour of the cosmetics industry, there's always the danger that the products we think are safe to put on our skin, might in actuality not be as safe as we think.

After studying the cosmetics industry, the truth is that these products have some of the largest mark-ups of any you're likely to find on the high street or in the mall! Your favorite face cream that cost you $80 may well have only cost as little as $2 to make, while that trendy lipstick you paid $30 of your hard-earned money for may actually only have a monetary value of $0.75! If you've bought thousands of dollars worth of cosmetics over the years, this realization can be pretty depressing. It doesn't feel good to know that all this time we've been duped by the cosmetics industry via slick marketing campaigns, while they made massive profits out of us unsuspecting consumers.

This is certainly something I've been a victim of. In the past, one of the things I would regularly spend money on was a good (and very expensive!) lipstick. Whenever I was having a bad day, I would head down to my favorite store and treat myself to a new shade. My friends would easily be able to tell if I was having a good year or not by the number of lipsticks I had in my collection! In hindsight, knowing what I know now, I feel a real sense of regret that I didn't get around to making my own cosmetics earlier. If I had of done, my bank balance certainly would have been a little healthier, and that money could have been better put to use.

The thing about the cosmetics industry is that even if you have a suspicion you're being ripped-off, it just feels that buying these products is something you *have to do*. I know a lot of women who would gladly fork over an inordinate amount of money for an excellent foundation! Why? Because you simply can't put a price on the confidence that looking your best can give you. The marketing used to sell cosmetic products has preyed on the insecurities of women for far too long. We are constantly bombarded with the message that if you want to feel good about yourself you need to look like a cover model; the implication being that the only way you'll be able to do that is to use their (expensive!) cosmetics. It's even gotten to the point where some women consider certain brands of makeup to be status symbols, much like they may do with a pair of expensive shoes or a designer handbag.

Am I immune to the marketing hype surrounding cosmetics? Honestly, no. I confess that even after learning the heartbreaking truth about the beauty industry I still get excited when I'm in the store browsing the makeup department. I still look at each lipstick color and eye shadow shade and imagine how I would incorporate them to achieve all sorts of glamorous looks. The only difference now is I don't purchase anywhere near as many products as I used to. These days I usually just look around in search of color inspiration, make a mental note and then create my own cosmetics at home. If you're thinking that the only reason I do this is to save a few dollars, you're wrong. Unfortunately there's more to it than that.

Harmful Ingredients Abound!

One of the sad realities when it comes to cosmetics is that the vast majority contain toxic ingredients. Even makeup products labeled as "all-natural" often times contain ingredients that may increase susceptibility to skin allergies, cancer, infertility and reproductive problems. If you're not sure about which ingredients you'd be best to avoid, here's a list of chemical nasties which are often used in cosmetics. Considering that human skin absorbs almost 60% of what is applied to it, this list will make you think twice next time you're about to splurge on expensive cosmetics.

- **Coal Tar** – Although already banned in the EU and Southeast Asia, there are still some products being sold in the US that contain this carcinogen. It's often found in treatments for dry skin as well as in anti-dandruff shampoos. Coal tar is also known as FD&C Red No.6.

- **Ethoxylated surfactants and 1,4-dioxane** – Created when carcinogenic ethylene oxide is added to a cocktail of other chemicals. This nasty toxin is found in some cosmetics, and unfortunately, is commonly found in baby washes being sold in the US. As a general rule, if you want to err on the safe side, avoid ingredients that contain the syllable "eth".

- **Fragrance/"Parfum"** – A catchall for unknown chemicals like phthalates. Fragrance has been proven to cause dizziness, headaches, asthma, and even allergic reactions in some unsuspecting victims.

- **Formaldehyde** – A proven irritant and likely carcinogen that can be found in hair dye, nail products, and shampoos. It is already banned in the EU.

- **Lead** – A carcinogenic contaminant found in most lipsticks and hair dyes. Since it's not officially considered to be an ingredient, you'll never see this listed on any beauty product.

- **Hydroquinone** – An ingredient used to peal and lighten skin. It is banned in the UK due to the fact it's been linked to cancer and reproductive disorders.

- **Mineral oil** – This petroleum byproduct can be found in moisturizers, baby oils, and styling gels.

- **Mercury** – An allergen that is known to impair brain function and development. Can be found in select eye drops and mascaras.

- **Parabens** – Used to preserve ingredients in many beauty and baby products. Has been linked to cancer, reproductive disorders, and endocrine problems.

- **Oxybenzone** – A chemical sunscreen that accumulates in fat cells. It can cause allergic reactions and hormone irregularity.

- **Phthalates** – A type of plasticizer that is banned in the EU and just recently, in California. It can be found in perfumes, deodorants, and lotions; and has been linked to kidney, liver, and lung damage.

- **Paraphenylenediamine (PPD)** – Present in hair dyes and styling products. Proven to be toxic to skin and can cause complications with the immune system.

- **Silicone derived emollients** – An ingredient added to some cosmetic products to make them feel soft. It has been linked to skin irritation and tumor enlargement.

-

- **Talc** – Has a similar composition to asbestos. Can be found in some blushes, eye shadows, baby powders, and deodorants. Has been linked to respiratory problems and ovarian cancer.

- **Sodium lauryl (ether) sulphate (SLS, SLES)** – An ingredient added to soap to make it foamy. It's easily absorbed by the body and can lead to irritation of sensitive skin.

- **Triclosan** – Can be found in some hand sanitizers, deodorants, and antibacterial products. It has been linked to endocrine disorders and cancer.

-

- **Toluene** – Has been linked to endocrine and

immune disorders. Often found in hair and nail products, this ingredient is often hidden under the term, "fragrance."

Check out the rest of "Homemade Makeup: A Complete Beginner's Guide To Natural DIY Cosmetics You Can Make Today" by Jane Aniston on Amazon.

Check Out My Other Books!

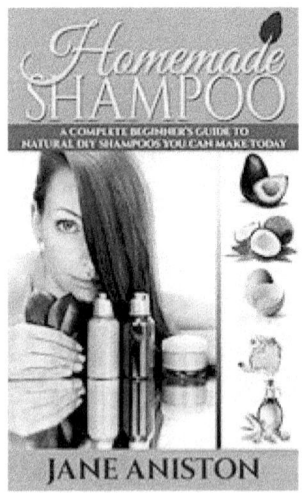

Homemade Shampoo (Includes 34 Organic Shampoo Recipes!)

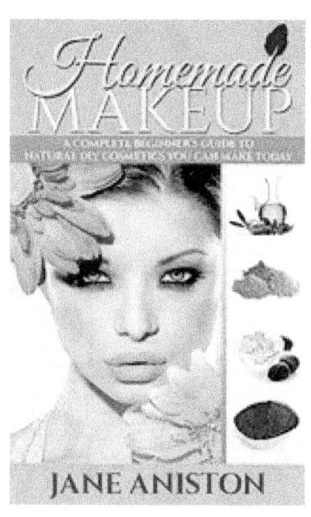

Homemade Makeup (Includes 28 Organic Makeup Recipes!)

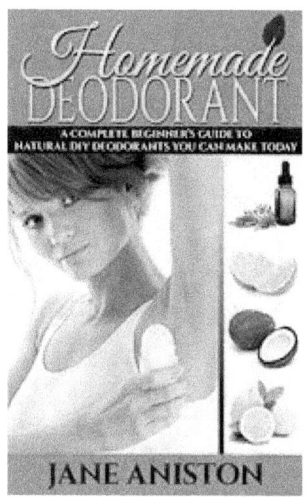

Homemade Deodorant (Includes 20 Organic Deodorant Recipes!)

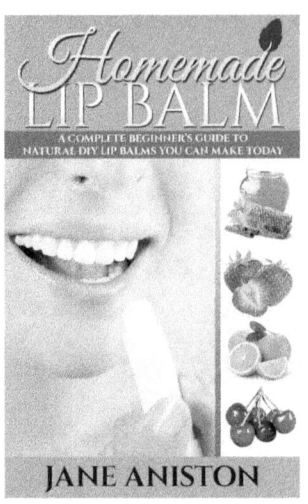

Homemade Lip Balm (Includes 22 Organic Lip Balm Recipes!)

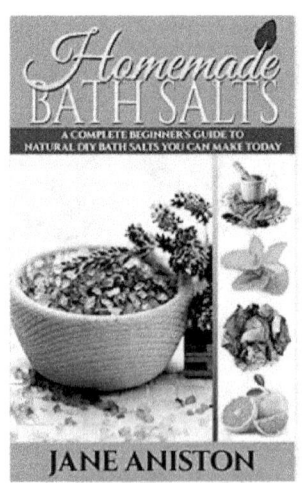

Homemade Bath Salts (Includes 35 Organic Bath Salt Recipes!)